Nootropics: Unlocking Your True Potential With Smart Drugs

First Edition, 2017

Copyright © 2017 The Nootropics Zone

Nootropics
Unlocking Your True Potential
With Smart Drugs

Nootropics

Table Of Contents

Disclaimer

The information contained in this book is for general information purposes only. While we've endeavored to keep the information up to date and correct, we make no representations or warranties of any kind, express or implied, about the completeness, accuracy, reliability, suitability or availability with respect to the book or the information, products, services, or related graphics contained in the book for any purpose. Any reliance you place on such information is therefore strictly at your own risk.

None of the statements made in this book have been reviewed by the Food and Drug Administration. The products and supplements mentioned in this book are not intended to diagnose, treat, cure, alleviate or prevent any diseases. All information in this book is the opinion of its respective authors who do not claim or profess to be medical professionals providing medical advice. This book is strictly for the purpose of providing opinions of the author. You should consult with your doctor or another qualified health care professional before you start taking any dietary supplements or engage in mental health programs. Any and all trademarks, logos brand names and service marks displayed in this book are the registered or unregistered Trademarks of their respective owners.

No part of this book may be reproduced or transmitted in any form or by any means, electronic or mechanical, including photocopying, recording or by any information storage and retrieval system, without written permission from the publisher.

Introduction

Do you want to have more focus, motivation, and energy?

Would you like to optimize the way your brain functions?

Are enhanced memory, reduced anxiety, improved mood, and increased concentration what you're looking for?

If you answered yes to any or all of these questions, then this book is definitely for you!

Over the past several years, interest in nootropics has been exploding. More and more people are using nootropics to increase focus, motivation, and energy, improve memory, and to reduce anxiety and depression. These wonderful substances are being used all over the world by people from every conceivable background. Doctors, lawyers, politicians, artists, musicians, businessmen (and women), computer programmers, students, and factory workers are all benefiting from using nootropics. And now, so can you!

If you're new to the wonderful world of nootropics, you'll have all the info you need to start benefiting from these amazing substances by the time you finish reading this book. And if you're already an experienced nootropic user, there's still a lot you'll learn from reading this. We've done our best to put together a book that is easy to understand for beginners, yet still informative for experienced users.

Thank you for reading!

Mike L.
The Nootropics Zone

CHAPTER ONE

What Are Nootropics?

What is a nootropic?

A nootropic is a supplement, plant, drug, vitamin, mineral, herb, amino acid, or other substance that improves at least one aspect of mental function. Examples of mental functions that nootropics can improve are memory, motivation, attention, focus, anxiety, mood, learning, and creativity.

By most definitions, a substance is only considered to be a nootropic if it improves cognitive function without causing any major side effects. Cocaine, for example, increases motivation, attention, focus, mood, and wakefulness. However, it is highly addictive and its use can have both acute and long-term health consequences. For these reasons, cocaine is not considered a nootropic.

Why do people use them?

Nootropics are used for a variety of reasons. Many people use them to boost cognitive performance and increase productivity. Others use them for their mood-boosting and anxiety-reducing effects. Some people find that certain nootropics work better than prescription medications for treating things like depression, anxiety, learning disorders, and ADHD.

The one thing that all nootropic users have in common is that they're trying to improve cognitive function. Some may be trying to increase focus without affecting mood. Others may be trying to reduce anxiety while improving memory. Everyone's goals are different, but the end result is the same: Improved overall cognitive performance.

The two reasons that people seem to use nootropics the most are for school and for work. Students use nootropics to help get homework done, study for exams, and pay attention in class. And nootropics are becoming increasingly popular in the workplace, especially among professionals. Doctors, lawyers, politicians, writers, artists, leaders in business, pilots, cooks, factory workers, shift workers, and computer programmers all use nootropics to stay on top of their game.

Here is a list of the most common reasons that people use nootropics:

- Increase focus
- Increase motivation
- Improve memory
- Improve learning
- Reduce anxiety
- Improve mood
- Treat various medical/mental disorders
- Improve overall cognition
- Increase creativity
- Increase logical thinking/problem solving

Do they actually work?

Yes! Many people are skeptical when they first hear about nootropics. But once they see for themselves how well they work, those skeptics are turned into believers.

It's important to understand that everyone's brain chemistry is different. Most people have to try a few different nootropics before they find the one or ones that work best for them. But they do work, absolutely.

There's plenty of research to show that they're effective. And on top of that, there are thousands of case reports around the internet of people's lives being changed for the better from taking nootropics. If the first one you try doesn't work for you, don't get discouraged. Since everyone's brain chemistry is different, not every nootropic will work the same way for everyone. Keep trying different nootropics and you're sure to find one that provides all the benefits you're looking for.

Can smart drugs really make you smarter?

Not exactly. However, they can improve your ability to learn, memorize information, recall information, focus your attention, and stay motivated.

While the use of nootropics will not increase your intelligence directly, they will improve your ability to engage in intellectual activity.

Over time, the use of nootropics could result in an increase in intelligence, if you spend your time engaged in intellectual activity. This has not been studied scientifically yet, but it makes sense theoretically. If you brain is primed to learn then, over time, you should become smarter if you dedicate yourself to learning new things or performing new tasks.

How to pronounce "nootropic"

The proper pronunciation of the word *nootropic* sounds like this: nO-ah-trO-pic.

However, most people pronounce it like this: new-trO-pic or new-traw-pic.

There's no right or wrong way to pronounce nootropic. Language is constantly evolving and the way words are pronounced often changes over time. But if you're a stickler for proper pronunciation, the first way is how the word was originally pronounced.

Origin of the word "nootropic"

The word *nootropic* was first coined by Dr. Corneliu Giurgea in 1972. Dr. Giurgea was a Romanian psychologist and chemist. He created the word nootropic out of the Greek words νους (mind), *nous* (intelligence), and τρέπειν (to bend or change).

Dr. Giurgea discovered the drug piracetam in 1964. Piracetam was the first racetam (see Chapter 3) ever created and inspired the creation of the term "nootropic." According to Dr. Giurgea, nootropics should have the following characteristics:

- They enhance learning and memory
- The protect the brain against physical and chemical injuries
- They enhance resistance to conditions that disrupt learned behaviors

- They increase the efficacy of the tonic cortical/subcortical control mechanisms
- They have few side effects and low toxicity

What are some other names for nootropics?

Nootropics have been called by a number of other names. Here are some of them:

- Smart drugs
- Cognitive enhancers
- Brain supplements
- Brain drugs
- Intelligence enhancers
- Mood brighteners
- Memory enhancers
- Neuro enhancers
- Nutraceuticals
- Brain pills
- Study aides
- Noots

Some people refer to them simply as *noots*, which is just a shortened version of the word *nootropics*. Typically, it's pronounced like this: newts.

How long have people been using them?

It's impossible to answer this question precisely. As long as modern humans have existed, they've tried to enhance their mental abilities through a variety of means. Plants, drugs, meditation, fasting, religious practices, sensory deprivation, and breathing techniques are just some of the ways that people have tried to improve their cognitive abilities throughout history.

Stimulants like caffeine and cocaine have been used for centuries to increase focus, motivation, attention, wakefulness, and memory. Opiates like morphine, heroin, and opium have been used for a long time to improve overall mood, relieve stress, and reduce anxiety.

Of course, most of these drugs would not be considered nootropics because of their well-known side effects. But it shows that people have an innate desire to improve the way they think and feel.

As far as modern nootropics go, we can get a more accurate look at when they were first used. Piracetam (see Ch. 4), the first in a class of nootropics called racetams to be created, was first synthesized in 1964. It became commercially available in the early 1970's. Since then, dozens of racetams have been created and many of them are used for their nootropic benefits. Other nootropic categories are even more modern. Eugeroics (see Ch. 3), like modafinil and adrafinil, were first created in the 1960's, but didn't start being used as nootropics until the 1990's.

Modern nootropics, like racetams and eugeroics, have only been used for the past few decades. But, people have been using plants and drugs to improve cognitive function all throughout history. Over the last 10 years or so, nootropic use has dramatically increased.

CHAPTER TWO

How Do Nootropics Work?

Neurotransmitters

Nootropics work by changing the levels of certain chemicals in the brain and the way that those chemicals interact with each other. These chemicals are called neurotransmitters. Neurotransmitters are responsible for mood, anxiety, focus, motivation, appetite, memory, libido, pleasure, pain, and anything else you can think of. They play a crucial role in what makes you, you.

By changing levels of specific neurotransmitters in the brain, we can change the way we think and feel. Take motivation, for example. We know that the neurotransmitter dopamine plays an important role in motivation. Generally, more dopamine means more motivation. Less dopamine, less motivation. So, taking a nootropic that increases dopamine in certain parts of the brain will lead to increased motivation.

This, of course, is a huge oversimplification. Brain chemistry is incredibly complex and modern science is only starting to scratch the surface of how the brain works. But we know that by taking nootropics, we can change the levels of neurotransmitters in the brain. And changing these levels will lead to changes in the way we think and feel.

What are neurotransmitters?

Neurotransmitters are chemicals produced naturally in the body that allow neurons to communicate with each other. When one neuron (nerve cell) needs to communicate with another neuron, it releases neurotransmitters in a junction called a synapse. Those neurotransmitters then bind to the receptors of the receiving neuron, sending the "message" from one neuron to the next.

Sound complicated? That's because it is. Neurotransmission is an incredibly complicated process and one that's far from being fully understood. It's only been in the past 100 years that we've known about this interesting process. And it's only been within the past few decades that we've had the technology to study how neurotransmitters work in the brain.

The first neurotransmitter to be discovered and identified was acetylcholine. It was discovered in 1915, but not in the brain – it was discovered in the heart. Acetylcholine is one of the neurotransmitters that several nootropics work on, so it's the perfect place to start.

Some key neurotransmitters affected by nootropics

Acetylcholine

As mentioned above, acetylcholine was the first neurotransmitter to be discovered. At the time, it was found to affect heart tissue. We now know that it does a lot more.

Acetylcholine has important functions in the central nervous system (CNS) and the peripheral nervous system (PNS). In the PNS, it works by activating muscle tissue. In the CNS, acetylcholine is known to play a role in memory, learning, arousal, and reward.

Low levels of acetylcholine in certain parts of the brain have been associated with brain fog, poor memory, and difficulty learning. Supplementing with cholinergics can increase levels of acetylcholine in the body and brain.

Cholinergics are things that increase acetylcholine levels in the body and brain. They are a popular class of nootropics (see Ch. 3) because they work well with other nootropics and they rarely have any side effects.

Popular cholinergic nootropics include:

- Alpha-GPC
- CDP-Choline (citicoline)
- Centrophenoxine
- Choline Bitartrate

Some nootropics, especially racetams like piracetam and oxiracetam, can cause headaches in some people. It is thought that this is due to low levels of acetylcholine in the brain. Taking a cholinergic with them usually eliminates the headaches.

Having adequate acetylcholine levels in the brain is necessary for optimal brain function. Taking a cholinergic nootropic ensures that your levels are where you want them to be.

Serotonin

Of all the neurotransmitters, this one is probably the most well-known. Serotonin (5-Hydroxytryptamine or 5-HT) is a neurotransmitter that is known to play a role in mood, appetite, sleep, and general well-being.

It's well-known because of drugs like Prozac (fluoxetine), Zoloft (sertraline), and Paxil (paroxetine). These drugs are antidepressants and are in a class called SSRI's – selective serotonin reuptake inhibitors. SSRI's work by changing the way serotonin acts in the synapse. To explain it simply, SSRI's cause serotonin to stay in the synapse longer, giving it a better chance to bind to the receptors of the target neuron.

Low levels of serotonin are commonly found in people that suffer from depression. That's why it was thought that depression is caused by low serotonin. The medical and scientific community are now starting to realize that depression is much more complicated than that. Though serotonin may play some role in depression, it's certainly not the whole story.

Several nootropics work by either increasing serotonin levels in the body or by changing the way serotonin works in the brain.

Popular serotonergic nootropics include:

- 5-HTP (5-Hydroxytryptophan)
- Rhodiola Rosea

While it doesn't play as large a role in learning, memory, and motivation as some other neurotransmitters, increasing serotonin levels in the brain can have indirect nootropic effects. Improving mood and feelings of well-being often result indirectly in increased motivation, focus, and memory.

Dopamine

Dopamine (short for 3,4 dihydrophenethylamine) is an important neurotransmitter that is associated with motivation, pleasure, libido, energy, and focus. Most addictive drugs, from alcohol to cocaine, affect dopamine in some way.

Some drugs, like cocaine, work on dopamine in much the same way that SSRI's work on serotonin. Cocaine is a dopamine reuptake inhibitor, leaving dopamine in the synapse longer, giving it more time to bind to the receptors of the neighboring neuron. Other drugs, called agonists, work by binding directly to dopamine receptors. Lastly, some drugs work simply by increasing dopamine levels throughout the brain.

Low dopamine levels are associated with lack of energy, lack of enjoyment (anhedonia), low sex drive (low libido), and decreased motivation. Some newer antidepressants work by targeting dopamine receptors in the brain. There are also older antidepressants, called MAOI's (monoamine oxidase inhibitors), that work by increasing dopamine levels. Unfortunately, they affect the levels of other monoamines (the class of neurotransmitters dopamine is in) and have tons of side effects.

There are several nootropics that either increase dopamine levels or bind directly to dopamine receptors. They are used to increase motivation, focus, creative thinking, and energy levels.

Popular dopaminergic nootropics include:

- Mucuna pruriens
- Adrafinil
- L-Tyrosine

GABA (gamma-aminobutyric acid)

Gamma-AminoButyric Acid, or GABA for short, is the primary inhibitory neurotransmitter in humans. It is associated with anxiety, sleep, relaxation, and other functions throughout the body and brain.

Several classes of anxiolytic (anti-anxiety) drugs affect GABA. Benzodiazepines and barbiturates are two examples of this. Newer drugs like Neurontin (gabapentin) and Lyrica (pregabalin) also work by affecting GABA, either directly or indirectly. Though only FDA approved for a few specific disorders, doctors have used these two drugs off-label to successfully treat dozens of different conditions. Some of the things these GABAergic drugs are being used to treat include generalized anxiety, OCD, restless leg syndrome, social anxiety, various phobias, bipolar disorder, depression, and several other disorders.

There are a number of nootropics that work by affecting GABA in the brain. They are generally the ones that reduce anxiety and promote feelings of well-being.

Some GABAergic nootropics include:

- L-Theanine
- Aniracetam
- Picamilon
- Sulbutiamine

These are just a few of the neurotransmitters that nootropics can affect. Over 60 neurotransmitters have been identified and it's possible that there are several more. But, the ones mentioned above are some of the most important neurotransmitters when it comes to nootropics.

How long do nootropics take to work?

This totally depends on the nootropic being used. Some start to work quickly, with the effects being felt within minutes. Others can takes weeks before any of the benefits are noticeable.

Many nootropics have both immediate and long-term benefits. Some of the effects are noticeable within an hour, but others don't become so for several weeks. One example of this would be phenylpiracetam (see Ch. 4). Users often notice an increase in motivation and focus after a single dose. However, it's not until several weeks of daily use that the memory-enhancing and other benefits of phenylpiracetam are realized.

Another thing that affects how long a nootropic takes to work is the route of administration (ROA). Nootropics can be taken in a variety of ways, just like other drugs and supplements. Some ROAs get whatever nootropic your taking into the bloodstream faster than others.

The vast majority of nootropics in this book work best when taken by mouth, orally. Other ROAs include intranasal (through the nose), sublingual (under the tongue), and inhalation. There are some drugs with nootropic properties that can be injected either intravenously (into the vein) or intramuscularly (into the muscle), but these ROAs are rarely used.

One example of a nootropic that can be administered safely and effectively by multiple ROAs is Noopept. Noopept is most commonly taken orally, by mouth. When taken this way, the effects are usually felt within an hour or so. But, Noopept can also be taken sublingually and intranasally. When taken sublingually, the effects are usually noticeable within 30 minutes. And, when taken intranasally, they are noticeable within minutes.

Generally, when it comes to ROA, intravenously administered drugs are felt first. This should come as no surprise, as they're injected directly into the bloodstream. Intranasal is next, followed by sublingual and lastly orally. Drugs that are taken by mouth have to be broken down and processed before they reach the bloodstream. And, if your stomach is filled with food, it usually takes even longer for the effects to be felt.

Do nootropics have side effects?

Side effects from most nootropics are rare. But, like all drugs and supplements, nootropics can potentially have side effects. These can range from a mild headache to a full-blown allergic reaction.

By some definitions, nootropics should not have any serious side effects. And most nootropics seem to be pretty safe for most people. But, like anything you put in your body, they can have unwanted effects.

Some of the more common potential side effects can include:

- Headaches
- Anxiety
- Insomnia
- Irritability

Allergic reactions are very rare, but can potentially happen. This is true not only of nootropics but of anything you put in your body. Any time you eat, drink, or even touch anything new, there's a risk that you'll have an allergic reaction. Though highly unlikely, it's always possible.

Different nootropics have different safety profiles. Some have been extensively studied and shown to be extremely safe. Others, especially some newer nootropics, haven't been studied as much and may have long-term side effects that are currently unknown. It's always important to do your research before putting anything new in your body. You can't make an informed decision about whether the potential risks are worth it if you aren't aware of those risks in the first place.

If you experience any minor side effects like a mild headache or insomnia, you should discontinue whatever is causing it. Side effects usually go away on their own as soon as you stop taking whatever was causing it. If your symptoms persist for a long period of time or get worse, consult a licensed physician. And, though very unlikely, if you have an allergic reaction (trouble breathing, extreme anxiety/panic, rapid heartbeat, severe rash), seek professional medical help immediately.

Are they addictive?

Anything that changes they way you think and feel can be addictive. There have been reports of people getting addicted to certain nootropics. However, these reports are rare and are usually only seen in people that already have problems with addiction.

Most drugs and supplements that are considered nootropics do not produce significant tolerance and withdrawal upon cessation. These characteristics are commonly associated with addictive drugs. There are exceptions, however. Stimulants like caffeine and amphetamines, which both have nootropic properties, are known to produce withdrawal symptoms after prolonged use.

Generally, nootropics are not addictive, but there are exceptions. Make sure you do your research before starting anything new. And know yourself: If you have a history of addictive behavior, you should use caution.

Will nootropics show up on a drug test?

This is a tricky question. The simple answer is no, they shouldn't. But false positives do happen and they happen a lot more than you might think.

A false positive is when a drug screen comes back positive for something that was never taken. Drug screens don't test for the drugs directly. They test for the metabolites that drugs break down into in the body. Sometimes unrelated drugs break down into similar metabolites causing a false reading.

Common drug screens do not look for nootropics. Standard 5-panel drug screens (commonly used for employment) only test for THC (cannabis), PCP, cocaine, amphetamines, and opiates.

Nootropics should not cause a false positive for any of these things. However, it's always possible. If you have to undergo extensive drug testing, it's recommended that you use caution.

And it should also be noted that amphetamines (Adderall, Vyvanse, Dexedrine, etc.) *will* show up on a standard drug screen. If you have a prescription for one of these medications, then it should not be a problem. Otherwise, you should not take any drugs containing any amphetamines.

Can you drink alcohol while taking a nootropic?

This is a broad question, as each nootropic works differently. The broad answer is no, you probably shouldn't.

Alcohol affects just about every system of the body, including the brain and the rest of the central nervous system. Nootropics work, at least in part, by changing the levels of certain chemicals in the brain. Mixing the two could cause unwanted side effects.

Some nootropics that have been extensively studied and are prescribed in some European countries have alcohol consumption warnings. Piracetam, for example, comes with the warning that you should not consume alcohol while taking it.

It's always good to err on the side of caution. It's probably not harmful to have a few drinks with most nootropics. But be aware, there could be some interactions.

What about cannabis?

Nootropics are drugs that improve memory, focus, attention, and motivation. Cannabis, for most people, has the exact opposite effect. By using cannabis with nootropics, you might be canceling out some of the cognition-enhancing effects.

That being said, mixing cannabis with certain nootropics can enhance other effects. Nootropics that affect mood and anxiety levels are often used with cannabis to increase their mood-boosting and anxiety-reducing effects.

Although the use of cannabis and nootropics together has not been scientifically studied, there's no reason to think that this combination would be dangerous.

So, yes, you probably can safely use cannabis and nootropics together. This combo may increase the anti-anxiety and antidepressant effects of some nootropics. However, it may also diminish some of the cognition-boosting effects.

CHAPTER THREE

The Different Types Of Nootropics

Classifying nootropics

Classifying drugs, supplements, or anything else that affects the body and brain can be a difficult task. There are a number of ways that you can organize them: By the effects they have, their chemical makeup, the neurotransmitters they affect, popularity of use, safety profile, effectiveness, etc.

We're gonna break them down into a few different categories that you're likely to see used in other books and around the internet. It can be a bit confusing, as some are categorized by their chemical makeup (racetams), others by their effects (eugeroics, adaptogens), and others by the way they work in the body (stimulants, precursors, cholinergics).

These are the categories that are most commonly used to classify nootropics. Let's look at the different categories and see what nootropics fall into each of them.

Racetams

The racetams are a well-known type of nootropic. In fact, it was the creation of the first racetam - piracetam - that inspired the creation of the word *nootropic*. You may recall from chapter 1 that it was the Romanian chemist and psychologist Corneliu Giurgea that first created piracetam in 1964. Since then, dozens of racetams have been created. Many of them have been studied and shown to have nootropic properties.

What all racetams have in common is that they all share a similar chemical backbone with a pyrrolidone nucleus. They are all based off of the first racetam, piracetam. While the effects of the racetams vary from one to another, several of them are known to influence the neurotransmitters acetylcholine and glutamate.

Each racetam has a different set of nootropic benefits. Some, like aniracetam, improve memory and reduce anxiety. Others, like phenylpiracetam and oxiracetam, act as mild stimulants. Most of the racetams that have been studied seem to improve at least one aspect of mental functioning.

Some nootropics, like Noopept and sunifiram, are often categorized as racetams because they are derived from them. However, they are not technically racetams, as they do not share a pyrrolidone nucleus.

Examples of racetams:

- Piracetam
- Aniracetam
- Oxiracetam
- Pramiracetam
- Phenylpiracetam

- Coluracetam
- Nefiracetam

It's very common in the world of drugs to group similar compounds together with the same suffix. As you can see, all the racetams end with the letters -tam.

Cholinergics

Cholinergics are another type of nootropic. These are compounds that increase levels of choline or acetylcholine in the brain. Acetylcholine is a neurotransmitter that is known to play a role in memory, motivation, focus, and muscle activation.

Cholinergics can increase levels of acetylcholine in the brain two different ways. They can either increase the levels directly by creating more acetylcholine, or increase them indirectly by preventing existing acetylcholine from breaking down.

It is common for nootropics users to stack (ch. 5) a cholinergic with one or more racetams. There are two reasons for doing this. First, several racetams are known to work (at least in part) by influencing acetylcholine in the brain. By taking a cholinergic, you increase your level of acetylcholine in the brain, thus enhancing the effects of taking a racetam.

The second reason for taking a cholinergic with a racetam is that it may reduce or eliminate certain side effects. Though uncommon, some people experience headaches and other side effects when taking a racetam. It is thought that these side effects are caused by low levels of acetylcholine. Taking a cholinergic increases acetylcholine levels, thus reducing or eliminating the headaches.

Examples of cholinergics:

- Alpha-GPC
- CDP-Choline (citicoline)
- Choline
- Centrophenoxine
- Huperzine-A

Eugeroics

This is a relatively new class of drugs. Eugeroics are drugs or other substances that promote wakefulness. They are used clinically to treat sleeping disorders, narcolepsy, excessive daytime sleepiness, and other conditions.

Eugeroics are very popular in the nootropics community. They share many of the same benefits as stimulants, but without most of the side effects. These benefits can include increased alertness, wakefulness, focus, motivation, and improved mood.

As of right now, there are only 3 drugs in this category: modafinil, armodafinil, and adrafinil. The first two are prescription drugs in the United States, used to treat narcolepsy, shift work sleep disorder, and excessive daytime sleepiness. Adrafinil is not a prescription drug in the U.S.

Examples of eugeroics:

- Adrafinil
- Armodafinil
- Modafinil

Adaptogens/Nutraceuticals

Adaptogens are substances that help to stabilize the body and brain, especially when stressed. While each adaptogen is unique, they all affect several bodily systems. Not all adaptogens are nootropics. However, several adaptogens have potent nootropic properties.

Many adaptogens are plants and herbs. Some of them have been used in Ayurvedic medicine and other Eastern medical traditions for centuries. They have been used (to varying degrees of success) to treat dozens of different conditions, and also as a general healing tonic.

Some of the adaptogens that have nootropic effects have been studied scientifically and found to be effective. Bacopa monnieri is a good example of this. It has several studies showing that it can improve memory and reduce anxiety. Other adaptogens, however, need more research before it can be definitively stated that they have nootropic properties.

Examples of adaptogens:

- Ashwagandha
- Bacopa monnieri
- Mucuna pruriens
- Ginseng
- Rhodiola rosea
- Gynostemma

Stimulants

Stimulants are substances that cause improvements in mental and/or physical functioning. Also called psychostimulants, this type of nootropic causes an increase in wakefulness, alertness, and motivation. Several stimulants are also known to improve mood and reduce the symptoms of depression.

It should be noted that, by some definitions, most stimulants are not true nootropics. This is because they can be habit forming and, over time, can lose their effectiveness. However, we are including them here because stimulants are widely used and unquestionably have nootropic properties.

The most commonly used stimulant is one that you may have already used today: caffeine. Not only is it the world's most used stimulant, but it's also the world's most used psychoactive drug. It has been extensively studied and is known to improve wakefulness, alertness, and other aspects of cognitive functioning.

Some of the more powerful stimulants are only available with a prescription. These include drugs like Adderall (mixed amphetamines), Vyvanse (lisdexamfetamine), Ritalin (methylphenidate), and Concerta (time-release methylphenidate). They are used to treat a number of conditions, including attention deficit-hyperactivity disorder (AD/HD), narcolepsy, and chronic fatigue syndrome.

These powerful stimulants all have several nootropic properties. Increased motivation, memory, focus, attention, and productivity are all commonly experienced when taking these drugs. Unfortunately, they can also come with a variety of side effects, including insomnia, tolerance, anxiety, restlessness, loss of appetite, and irritability.

Examples of stimulants:

- Caffeine
- Amphetamines (Adderall, Vyvanse, Desoxyn)
- Methylphenidate (Ritalin, Concerta)
- Nicotine
- Ephedrine

Precursors

This is another class of substances that isn't commonly thought of as being nootropic. However, these substances can all have significant nootropic effects.

Simply put, a precursor is a substance that converts into another substance in the body. Through a series of chemical reactions, precursors assist in the creation of different compounds in the body and brain.

Take serotonin, for example. Serotonin is a neurotransmitter that has several functions in the body and brain. It is known to play a role in mood, appetite, and sleep, among other things. The dietary supplement 5-HTP is a direct precursor to serotonin. In other words, our bodies use 5-HTP to create serotonin. So when we take 5-HTP, our bodies use it to create serotonin, resulting in a number of nootropic benefits. These benefits include improved mood and sleep.

Examples of precursors:

- L-Dopa
- L-Tyrosine
- L-Tryptophan

- 5-HTP
- Glutamine

Miscellaneous/Other

Most cognition-enhancing substances fit into one or more of the types of nootropics listed above. However, there are some that don't quite fit into any of those categories.

The nootropics (or substances with nootropic properties, we should say) that don't fit nicely into any of the types above come from all different classifications. Sulbutiamine, for example, is a variation of vitamin B1 (thiamine). L-theanine, on the other hand, is an amino acid. Neither of these substances really fit into any of the types of nootropics listed above. However, both of them have several nootropic properties.

Here are some examples of substances with nootropic properties that don't fit into any of the other categories:

- L-Theanine
- Sulbutiamine
- Uridine
- Vinpocetine
- Acetyl L-Carnitine (ALCAR)

CHAPTER FOUR

Common Nootropics

In this chapter, we're gonna take a look at some common nootropics that are being used around the world. This list could be much longer and if you're interested in learning about other nootropics, we discuss the best places to find information about smart drugs in chapter 7. But in this chapter, we're just gonna explore some of the most popular nootropics being used today.

This list is alphabetical and includes a variety of nootropics from every type. Most of these have been scientifically studied and shown to be both safe and effective. Some of them work best when taken in combination with other nootropics. This is called *stacking* and we'll go over it in chapter 5. Again, this isn't an all-inclusive list, but rather a list of the safest, most popular, and most effective nootropics.

Adrafinil

This is a powerful nootropic that is used for its ability to enhance wakefulness, increase focus, and improve mood. Adrafinil is a prodrug of modafinil, which means that it converts into modafinil once it's in the body. Because of this, it has all the same benefits of modafinil. However, higher doses are needed to experience its cognition-enhancing benefits.

Adrafinil boosts the neurotransmitter hypocretin. This neurotransmitter plays a role in appetite, arousal, and wakefulness. Increasing hypocretin is thought to increase levels of other important neurotransmitters, like dopamine, histamine, and norepinephrine.

We know that dopamine plays a crucial role in focus, motivation, learning, reward, pleasure, and energy. It's through the indirect increase in dopamine that adrafinil may exert its nootropic effects.

Other Names

- Olmifon
- CRL-40028

Type

- Eugeroic

Benefits

- Increased focus
- Increased productivity
- Increased alertness
- Increased motivation

Side Effects/Warnings

Adrafinil is generally well tolerated. Most users experience few side effects, if any. The most common side effects of adrafinil include headache, insomnia, nausea, and nervousness. Taking adrafinil early in the day may reduce the risk of having insomnia (difficulty sleeping).

Dosage

Adrafinil is typically dosed at anywhere from 300-900 milligrams (mg) once or twice a day. Most users report that they experience increased focus, wakefulness, and motivation from between 300-600 mg. Others say that they need 900 mg to feel adrafinil's effects. You should always start with a low dose and work your way up as needed. Most people find that 300 mg is a good starting point with adrafinil.

Every 300 mg of adrafinil you take converts into about 100 mg of modafinil once it passes through the liver. Modafinil is usually dosed between 100-300 mg, so it makes sense that adrafinil would be effective at doses ranging from 300-900 mg.

Unless you are taking adrafinil to stay awake overnight, it's recommended that you take it early in the day to avoid insomnia. And you should avoid taking adrafinil daily for long periods of time, as it can slightly raise liver enzymes. If you decide to stay on a eugeroic for more than a couple months, modafinil and armodafinil are better choices. Adrafinil seems to be safe for short-term use, but long-term use could come with an increase in side effects.

Alpha-GPC

This is a natural choline compound that's found in the brain. It's also a precursor to the neurotransmitter acetylcholine. As mentioned in chapter 2, acetylcholine is known to play a role in memory, motivation, muscle activation, and attention. Of all the known cholinergics, alpha-GPC raises acetylcholine levels the most effectively.

Alpha-GPC is taken to improve memory, motivation, learning, and overall cognitive enhancement. It's also frequently stacked with other smart drugs, as it can increase the effectiveness and reduce the potential side effects of certain nootropics. Most commonly, Alpha-GPC is taken with one or more racetams. They are known to cause headaches in some users and taking alpha-GPC with them can eliminate this side effect.

Used on its own or stacked with other smart drugs, alpha-GPC is a common nootropic that increases your brain's acetylcholine levels in a safe and effective manner.

Other Names

- L-Alpha Glycerylphosphorylcholine
- Choline Alfoscerate
- Glycerophosphocholine
- L-Alpha Glycerophosphocholin

Type

- Cholinergic

Benefits

- Improved learning
- Increased motivation
- Improved memory
- Improved physical performance
- Increased growth hormone (HGH) levels
- Faster reaction time
- Overall cognitive enhancement

Side Effects/Warnings

Alpha-GPC is extremely well-tolerated. Most users do not experience any side effects. When they do experience them, they are generally mild and go away as soon as supplementation is stopped.

Potential side effects can include headache, heartburn, insomnia, dizziness, skin rash, and confusion. They are rare and only affect a small percentage of users.

Dosage

Most of the studies done on alpha-GPC have use doses between 600 – 1,200 mg. At these doses, alpha-GPC has been found to be very safe and with few side effects.

For nootropic benefits, users usually take anywhere from 500 to 1,500 mg of alpha-GPC every day. This is usually taken in 2 or 3 divided doses throughout the day.

Alpha-GPC can be taken with or without food. It may absorb a little better when taken on an empty stomach. However, many users report that this causes heartburn and upset stomach. If this happens to you, taking alpha-GPC with a small meal may help to reduce or eliminate these side effects.

Aniracetam

Aniracetam is an ampakine nootropic that is a member of the racetam family. Unlike other racetams, aniracetam has been shown to have a powerful anxiolytic (anti-anxiety) effect in addition to providing a number of nootropic benefits. Like the other racetams, aniracetam exerts its nootropic effects by stimulating the AMPA receptor site in the brain. AMPA receptors are known to play a vital role in learning and memory.

What really makes aniracetam unique is its ability to reduce anxiety without causing sedation. This is caused, at least in part, by aniracetam's ability to stimulate dopamine and serotonin. As you may recall from chapter 2, dopamine is known to play a large role in motivation, focus, pleasure, and certain types of anxiety. Serotonin is strongly associated with mood, appetite, and sleep.

In the United States, aniracetam is sold legally as a dietary supplement. In several European countries, however, it is only available with a prescription.

Other Names

- Draganon
- Sarpul
- Ampamet
- Memodrin
- Referan
- N-anisoyl-2-pyrrolidinone
- 1-p-anisoyl-2-pyrrilidinone
- CAS 72432-10-1

Type

- Racetam

Benefits

- Reduced anxiety
- Increased focus
- Improved memory
- Improved learning ability
- Improved mood
- Improved cognitive processing

Side Effects/Warnings

Aniracetam is generally considered to be very safe. At recommended doses, side effects are rarely reported. The most common side effects reported are headache, nausea, and gastrointestinal problems. Fortunately, the nausea and gastrointestinal problems can usually be avoided by taking aniracetam with food.

Like the other racetams, aniracetam can increase the brain's demand for acetylcholine, which can lead to mild or moderate headaches. This can easily be avoided by taking aniracetam with a cholinergic, like alpha-GPC or CDP-choline. As an added bonus, stacking aniracetam with a cholinergic has been shown to increase the nootropic effects of aniracetam.

Dosage

Aniracetam is usually found to be effective at a dosage of anywhere from 750-2,500 mg a day, taken in 1-3 divided doses. Many users report great results with just 750 mg. Others require several times that for optimal results.

Aniracetam is fat soluble. For maximum absorption, it is recommended that you take it with a small meal that contains about 10 or 15 grams of fat. Though not necessary, this will help your body absorb more of this potent nootropic.

Ashwagandha

Ashwagandha is a common name for the plant *withania somnifera*. This is a plant with tons of health benefits. It has been used in Ayurvedic medicine for centuries to treat a number of different conditions and as a general healing tonic.

The word ashwagandha means "smell of horse." It was given this name for two reasons: First, the root has a distinct horse-like smell to it. Second, it has been used for centuries to increase virility, giving it the reputation of making you as strong as a horse.

Unlike many newer substances with nootropic properties, ashwagandha has been around for centuries and has a lot of research to support its safety and effectiveness. It's classified as an adaptogen because it helps the body fight stress and maintain a homeostatic balance.

In addition to having a number of nootropic benefits, Ashwagandha also has a number of physiological benefits. It's been extensively studied and shown to improve cholesterol levels, reduce blood pressure, heart rate, and cortisol levels, boost libido and sexual function, and increase testosterone/DHEA/LH levels in men. Ashwagandha is an amazing plant that has a ton of benefits and a long history of safe use.

Other Names

- Withania Somnifera
- Indian Ginseng
- Winter Cherry
- Dunal
- Solanaceae

Type

- Adaptogen

Benefits

- Decreased anxiety
- Improved mood
- Increased motivation
- Increased/improved social functioning
- Reduced social anxiety
- Reduced fatigue
- Improved cholesterol levels
- Reduced cortisol
- Increased testosterone/DHEA/LH
- Reduced blood pressure and heart rate
- Increased fertility/Libido
- Improved immune function

Side Effects/Warnings

Ashwagandha is very well-tolerated by most people. Side effects seem to be rare and easily reversible by simply stopping ashwagandha.

If you have an autoimmune disease, like Lupus, Crohn's, Multiple Sclerosis, Rheumatoid Arthritis, or others, it is theoretically possible that ashwagandha could make your condition worse. Ashwagandha can boost certain parts of the immune system and this could, in theory, lead to a flare up of your condition. However, this is all theoretical: We couldn't find a single instance of this happening in the medical literature.

Don't take ashwagandha if you are pregnant or nursing. If you are diabetic, you should know that ashwagandha can lower blood sugar levels. While this is often a desirable effect, be aware that it may interfere with some diabetic medications.

Ashwagandha can also irritate the gastrointestinal (GI) tract. You should not use it if you currently suffer from stomach ulcers.

Lastly, ashwagandha can cause upset stomach, nausea, and vomiting. These side effects are rare and can usually be reduced or eliminated by taking it with a small meal.

Dosage

Ashwagandha works best when taken two or three times a day, over the course of several weeks/months. Most of the benefits of ashwagandha will only be noticeable after several weeks of supplementation.

However, some effects are noticeable after one dose. A reduction in anxiety and a reduction in some of the symptoms of stress have been observed after one dose.

The lowest potentially effective ashwagandha dose is between 300-500 mg. If you are using ashwagandha to potentiate another anxiolytic (e.g., aniracetam) a smaller dose may be effective, possibly between 100-200 mg.

The optimal ashwagandha dosage is 6,000 mg every day. This is the dosage that has been shown to have the most benefits in several clinical studies. It should be taken in 3 divided doses of 2,000 mg each and it should be taken with food.

Bacopa Monnieri

Bacopa monnieri (often referred to simply as Bacopa) is a perennial herb that grows naturally all over the world. It's been used in Ayurvedic medicine for centuries to improve mental function and to treat a number of physical illnesses.

In modern times, Bacopa is used to reduce anxiety, improve memory, and as a general brain booster. It is sold in pill and powder form as a dietary supplement and is considered to be an adaptogen.

Bacopa is known to interact with the dopamine and serotonin neurotransmitter systems. If you recall from chapter 2, dopamine is known to play an important role in focus, memory, reward, pleasure, and anxiety. Serotonin is associated with mood, appetite, and sleep. Bacopa has been shown to promote communication between neurons. It increases the growth of nerve endings, enhancing the rate that the nervous system can communicate. It's also a potent antioxidant.

Other Names

- Brahmi
- Aindri
- Water hyssop
- Indian Pennywort
- Jalabrahmi
- Lysimachia monnieri L. Cent.
- Thyme-leafed gratiola

Type

- Adaptogen

Benefits

- Reduced anxiety
- Improved memory
- Promotes healthy neurotransmitter levels
- Increased focus
- Overall improvement in cognitive performance

Side Effects/Warnings

Most people that take Bacopa don't experience any side effects. For those that do, the most common side effect is upset stomach. This can usually be remedied by taking Bacopa with food.

If you are taking prescription antidepressants, you should talk to your doctor before taking Bacopa. An unlikely (yet potentially life-threatening) interaction called serotonin syndrome could occur. No known cases of serotonin syndrome have ever been reported with Bacopa. But, since it increases serotonin in the brain, it is theoretically possible.

Dosage

Bacopa doesn't work instantly. It may take several weeks before you notice the full benefits of supplementing with Bacopa. Many people do report an instant reduction in anxiety after their first dose. However, it can take several weeks before you notice the full benefits.

To reduce the possibility of upset stomach, you may want to take Bacopa with food. A good starting dosage for most people is 375 mg a day. If you don't notice any effect after a few weeks, you may want to consider increasing the dosage.

Caffeine

Even if you're brand new to the wonderful world of nootropics, there's a good chance you're familiar with this one. You might even have some of this in your system right now! Caffeine is the most widely used psychoactive drug and certainly the most commonly used nootropic. It's been used all over the world for centuries to increase wakefulness, boost mood, improve focus, and increase overall cognitive and physical performance.

Caffeine is a potent central nervous system stimulant and is categorized as such. Chemically, it's classified as a xanthine. Many of caffeine's benefits are due to it being an adenosine receptor antagonist. Adenosine receptors can cause relaxation and sedation when activated. Antagonists are substances that block or reduce the effects of neurotransmitters. As an antagonist, caffeine is able to block these effects, leading to feelings of stimulation and wakefulness.

Other Names

- Coffee extract
- Tea extract
- 1,3,7-trimethylxanthine
- Anhydrous caffeine
- Cafeina
- Trimethylxanthine
- 1,3,7-Trimethyl-1h-purine-2,6(3H,7H)-dione

Type

- Stimulant

Benefits

- Increased alertness
- Increased wakefulness
- Improved focus
- Improved mood
- Increased endurance

Side Effects/Warnings

Caffeine is generally regarded as safe (GRAS) when taken at recommended dosages. Side effects can include insomnia, nervousness, restlessness, upset stomach, nausea, vomiting, and increased heart rate. Caffeine may increase the effects of other stimulants.

Unlike most other nootropics, caffeine has the potential to be habit-forming. Over time, tolerance and addiction may occur. If you use caffeine daily for a long period of time, you may experience withdrawal if you stop using it abruptly. Withdrawal symptoms can include headache, anxiety, tiredness, irritability, and depression.

Dosage

Ideal caffeine dosages will vary greatly from person to person. A good starting point for most people that want to supplement with caffeine is 100 mg. This is roughly the equivalent of one large cup of coffee. Some people require significantly more for optimal effects. There have been a number of scientific studies that used up to 500 mg per dose and showed it to be generally safe.

To increase the effectiveness of caffeine, many nootropic users like to stack it with l-theanine. Taking caffeine and l-theanine together is extremely popular because it increases the benefits of each while, at the same time, reduces side effects. L-theanine eliminates the jitters, anxiety, and restlessness that caffeine can cause on its own. We'll explore this much more in chapter 5.

CDP-Choline

CDP-choline, also commonly called citicoline, is a nootropic with a number of physical and cognitive benefits. It's known to improve memory, attention, motivation, and other aspects of cognitive functioning.

Some of CDP-choline's benefits can be explained by its ability to convert to choline and uridine in the body. Once those substances cross the blood-brain-barrier, they convert back into CDP-choline, resulting in an increase in the neurotransmitter acetylcholine.

Another way that CDP-choline may exert some of its effects is through its ability to increase dopamine receptor densities in certain parts of the brain. This helps to explain, at least in part, how CDP-choline supplementation is able to improve motivation and attention.

Lastly, CDP-choline seems to increase levels of growth hormone (HGH), luteinizing hormone (LH), thyroid-stimulating hormone (TSH), and follicle-stimulating hormone (FSH), at least under some conditions. This mechanism of action may also help to explain some of CDP-choline's effects.

Other Names

- Citicoline
- Cytidine Diphosphate-Choline
- 5'-diphosphocholine
- Citicholine
- CDPC
- Citicolina
- Cytidine Diphosphocholine

Type

- Cholinergic

Benefits

- Improved memory
- Improved learning
- Increased attention
- Decreased appetite
- Increased motivation
- Increased acetylcholine

Side Effects/Warnings

CDP-choline has an excellent safety profile. Side effects are very rare and, when they do occur, they are usually very mild.

When side effects occur, they may include insomnia, headache, upset stomach, diarrhea, nausea, blurred vision, low or high blood pressure, and dizziness. If you experience any of these side effects, simply stop taking CDP-choline and they should resolve on their own.

Dosage

CDP-choline is usually taken at a dosage of anywhere from 500 to 2,000 mg a day. It can be taken all at once but may work best if taken in two divided doses, 8-12 hours apart.

As with all nootropics, it's recommended that you start with a low dosage and work your way up as needed. Some users report great results with just 500 mg a day. Others report that they don't notice any effects until they get up to 2,000 mg a day. It's generally recommended that you start with 250 mg twice a day for the first couple weeks and then increase the dose if you are not experiencing the desired results.

CDP-choline may absorb a little better when taken on an empty stomach. However, this is not necessary. If you experience nausea or upset stomach, you should take CDP-choline with a small meal.

Coluracetam

Of all the nootropics available today, coluracetam is one of the newest. It was first created in 2005 by Mitsubishi Tanabe, a Japanese pharmaceutical company. They first synthesized it by modifying the well-known nootropic piracetam.

Clinical trials are being conducted on coluracetam to investigate its usefulness at treating nervous system and eye disorders. So far, the research has been very promising. Findings from the clinical trials have suggested that coluracetam could be used to treat people who are diagnosed with both major depressive disorder (MDD) and generalized anxiety disorder (GAD).

Nootropic users have found that coluracetam provides a number of cognition-enhancing benefits. Many say that it significantly increases motivation, improves sensory experiences, reduces anxiety, and improves mood. Aside from the effects on depression and anxiety noted in the early clinical trials, none of the nootropic benefits of coluracetam have been scientifically demonstrated, yet.

Other Names

- BCI-540
- MKC-231
- 2-(2-oxopyrrolidin-1-yl)-N-(2,3-dimethyl-5,6,7,8-tetrahydrofuro2,3-b quinolin-4-yl)acetoamide

Type

- Racetam

Benefits

- Increased motivation
- Improved mood
- Reduced anxiety
- Enhanced sensory experience

Side Effects/Warnings

Coluracetam has not been extensively studied in humans. Much more research is necessary before it can be conclusively stated that it's safe.

However, in the studies that have been done on humans, coluracetam has been shown to be very safe. Researchers reported that after a daily coluracetam dosage of 240 mg in clinical trials, none of the participants had any serious side effects. This is the highest dosage that has been studied and shown to be safe, so far.

Dosage

Coluracetam is usually taken between 1 and 3 times a day in doses ranging from 5-40 mg. Some people report great results with a low dose. As with all nootropics, you should always start low and work your way up as needed.

The highest coluracetam dosage used in clinical trials was 80 mg taken 3 times a day. In that study, no serious side effects were reported at that dosage.

Ginkgo Biloba

Ginkgo biloba, often referred to simply as "ginkgo," is the most commonly used supplement for brain health. It's been used for thousands of years all over the world to treat a number of conditions. Ginkgo has a long history of use in traditional Chinese medicine and has been used for its health benefits by many other cultures.

In recent years, ginkgo biloba extract has been consumed for its nootropic benefits. Users report improved memory, reduced anxiety, increased reaction time, improved blood flow, and general cognitive enhancement, among other benefits.

Other Names

- Ginkgo
- Maidenhair Tree
- Tanakan
- Tebonin
- Rokan

Type

- Adaptogen

Benefits

- Improved memory
- Reduced anxiety
- Increased reaction time
- Overall cognitive enhancement

Side Effects/Warnings

Ginkgo biloba is generally very well-tolerated. Most people that take it do not experience any side effects. However, side effects are possible, just like with anything you put in your body.

Some of the most common side effects include upset stomach, headache, dizziness, and skin reactions. These side effects are usually mild and go away shortly after discontinuing ginkgo.

If you are taking prescription antidepressants, especially MAOI's, it is especially important that you talk to your doctor before taking ginkgo. If you have seizures, ginkgo may not be right for you, as it may make you more likely to have one. And lastly, you should not take ginkgo if you are pregnant or plan on becoming pregnant.

Dosage

Studies have used dosages from 120 mg a day and up. In the studies that compared the effectiveness of more than one dosage, the higher dosage usually showed greater results. Many users report the best results from a dosage of 500 mg per day, either once a day or divided into two doses.

Ginkgo extract can be taken with or without food. It may be slightly more effective if taken on an empty stomach. However, this can cause upset stomach in some people. If this happens to you, try taking ginkgo with a small meal. Most users like to take it early in the day.

L-Theanine

L-theanine, often referred to as just theanine, is an amino acid analogue of the amino acids L-glutamate and L-glutamine. It was first discovered in 1949 as a constituent of green tea. Unfortunately, you'd have to drink gallons and gallons of green tea to get the full benefits of theanine. By taking it as a supplement, you can experience all that it has to offer.

L-theanine is known to reduce mental stress, physical stress, anxiety, and improve mood. While theanine does work on its own, it's most commonly taken with caffeine. When taken together, theanine and caffeine work synergistically.

Taken on its own, caffeine is known to cause anxiety, jitters, and restlessness in some people, especially at high doses. Most people find that when taken with theanine, these caffeine side effects are greatly reduced or eliminated completely.

Other Names

- Theanine
- N-Ethyl-L-Glutamine
- L-gamma-glutamylethylamide
- 5-N-Ethyl-Glutamine

Type

- Misc/Other

Benefits

- Reduced mental stress
- Reduced physical stress

- Reduced anxiety
- Improved mood

Side Effects/Warnings

L-theanine has been shown to be extremely safe when taken on its own. When taken with caffeine, all the usual side effects of caffeine are possible, though theanine will likely reduce or eliminate some side effects.

The Food and Drug Administration (FDA) has granted theanine GRAS (generally recognized as safe) status. This means that there is a lot of evidence to support its safe use. Though side effects are very rare, they can occur. They are usually mild and may include headache, dizziness, and upset stomach.

Dosage

L-theanine has been shown to be safe in dosages as high as 1,200 mg per day. Most users experience the benefits of theanine with a dose between 100-400 mg. Even though it's known to be very safe, you should always start with a low dose and work up as needed.

When taken with caffeine, as it's commonly done, most users find that a 1:1 or a 2:1 ratio of theanine to caffeine is optimal. A good starting point would be 200 mg of theanine and 200 mg of caffeine, which is the dose that most caffeine pills come in. For people that are especially sensitive to caffeine, 100 mg of each might work better.

Modafinil

Modafinil is a drug that was first created in the 1970's. It didn't start to see widespread use until the late 1990's and early 2000's when it was approved by the FDA (under the brand name Provigil) to treat narcolepsy, shift work sleep disorder, and sleep apnea. Since then, modafinil has become increasingly popular as a treatment for other disorders and as a powerful nootropic.

Classified as a eugeroic, modafinil has been shown to increase wakefulness, reduce fatigue, improve cognition and memory, reduce reaction time, and even improve mood and motivation. With such an impressive list of positive effects, it should come as no surprise that modafinil is as popular as it is. Users all over the world have been enjoying its cognition-enhancing benefits for over a decade now.

Modafinil is closely related to the drug adrafinil. The effects of both are very similar, but they do have some important differences. Adrafinil is a prodrug of modafinil. What that means is that adrafinil converts into modafinil once it's ingested. Because of this, adrafinil takes longer for its effects to be felt and also requires a higher dosage. Most users that have tried both prefer modafinil because a lower dosage is required and the effects come on faster.

Other Names

- Provigil
- Modavigil
- Modvigil
- Alertec
- Modapro
- Alertex

- 2-[(Diphenylmethyl)sulfinyl]acetamide

Type

- Eugeroic

Benefits

- Improved cognitive performance
- Improved mood
- Increased memory
- Reduced fatigue
- Reduced reaction time
- Increased alertness
- Increased motivation

Side Effects/Warnings

Modafinil is generally well tolerated by most people. Most users find that the benefits outweigh any potential side effects. However, side effects can occur. They may include headaches, insomnia, nausea, anxiety, dizziness, and upset stomach. These side effects usually go away on their own after discontinuing modafinil. It is also possible that modafinil may interact with hormonal contraceptives.

Dosage

People that use modafinil for its nootropic benefits frequently find a dosage of anywhere from 100-400 mg a day to be effective. Most of the studies that have been done on modafinil used dosages within that range.

As always, you should start with a low dosage and work your way up as needed. For most people, 200 mg seems to be a good starting point. If you're particularly small or usually sensitive to drugs like modafinil, a starting dosage of 100 mg may work better.

It's also generally recommended that you take modafinil early in the day. Taking it later in the day may result in unwanted insomnia. If you're taking modafinil to stay awake or to combat sleep deprivation, this obviously won't be a problem.

Modafinil can be taken with or without food. Taking it on an empty stomach may help it to absorb better. This will make its effects come on sooner and stronger. For some people, taking it on an empty stomach may cause gastrointestinal discomfort. This can easily be remedied by taking modafinil with food, preferably a small meal.

Mucuna Pruriens

Mucuna pruriens is a tropical legume that grows naturally in several parts of Africa and Asia. It has been used for centuries to treat a number of different ailments in Eastern medicine – everything from snake bites to Parkinson's disease.

This interesting bean contains a number of different substances that are known to have physiological effects. The most significant is l-dopa, but mucuna also contains serotonin, 5-HTP, bufotenine, dimethyltryptamine (DMT), nicotine, beta carboline, and 5-MEO-DMT. It's unlikely that these have any noticeable effect, though, as they are only found in very small quantities.

In recent years, mucuna pruriens has become popular in nootropic and fitness communities. For many users, it provides a noticeable improvement in mood, increased motivation, and a reduction in anxiety. This makes it a great part of any nootropic stack or as a preworkout supplement. There is also some research to suggest that it may increase testosterone and growth hormone (HGH) levels.

Other Names

- Velvet bean
- Cowitch
- Cowage
- Lacuna bean
- Lyon bean
- Florida velvet bean
- Yokohama velvet bean
- Muritius velvet bean
- Bengal velvet bean

Type

- Adaptogen

Benefits

- Improved mood
- Increased sense of well-being
- Reduced anxiety
- Increased dopamine levels
- Possibly increased testosterone and HGH

Side Effects/Warnings

Mucuna seems to be very well tolerated when taken at recommended dosages. One large double-blind study showed that mucuna had no serious side effects at a dosage of 30 grams for 20 weeks.

Since mucuna pruriens contains l-dopa, the side effects of l-dopa are theoretically possible. However, several studies have shown that mucuna seems to have fewer side effects than l-dopa. This may be due to mucuna containing other substances in addition to l-dopa, which may mitigate certain side effects.

Some users report nausea, gastrointestinal distress, and upset stomach after taking mucuna. This can usually be eliminated by taking mucuna with food.

If you are taking an MAOI (typically prescribed for severe depression) or other psychiatric drugs that affect dopamine levels, you should talk to your prescriber before taking mucuna.

Dosage

The optimal mucuna dosage is going to depend on the percentage of l-dopa it contains. Unfortunately, there is a lot of variation between manufacturers. Some mucuna products have as little as 10% l-dopa, while others have as much as 98%.

If you are using a 98% l-dopa mucuna product, a good starting point would be 250 mg twice a day. Some acute effects may be noticeable within an hour or two of administration. However, the full benefits of mucuna are usually only seen after several weeks of supplementation.

If you don't experience the desired results at that dosage, you can increase the dosage as needed. It is recommended that you only increase the daily dosage of mucuna/l-dopa every 4-7 days and by no more than 750 mg at a time.

While there are no established guidelines for optimal mucuna dosing, there are guidelines for l-dopa. L-dopa is typically started at 250 mg twice a day and titrated (adjusted) slowly up to a maximum of around 6,000 mg a day.

Although the safety of taking high dose (>6,000 mg) l-dopa has been well-established, it is not needed to experience its nootropic benefits.

Mucuna is probably absorbed best when taken on an empty stomach. However, if you experience nausea and upset stomach, you should take mucuna with food.

Lastly, mucuna may work better when taken with epigallocatechin gallate (EGCG). EGCG, commonly found in green tea, is a decarboxylase inhibitor. By taking EGCG with mucuna, it helps to keep more dopamine in your central nervous system (brain). This increases the positive effects of mucuna/l-dopa and reduces the likelihood of side effects.

Noopept

Noopept is a peptide-derived smart drug that is very similar to nootropics in the racetam family, like aniracetam or piracetam. However, it is much more potent and has a higher bioavailability.

In the United States, Noopept is sold legally as a dietary supplement. In several European countries and in Russia, it is only available with a prescription. It has a number of benefits, including improved mood, reduced anxiety, and improved overall cognitive performance.

Although it is technically not in the same family as the racetams, it works in a similar way. Noopept works on NDMA and AMPA receptor sites and their pathways of function. It also has an affinity for the acetylcholine system. This goes a long way in explaining its nootropic effects.

Noopept has also been shown to have an anxiolytic (anxiety reducing) effect. This is thought to be caused by Noopept's ability to stimulate dopamine (specifically D2 and D3) receptor sites and Ach nicotinic receptor sites. Dopamine is known to play a crucial role in motivation, focus, pleasure, and anxiety. It may also stimulate certain serotonin receptors, which explains its mood-boosting effects.

Noopept is such a powerful nootropic that it is being investigated as a possible treatment for Alzheimer's Disease. It is thought that it may be able to repair damaged cells and receptor sites in the brain that are commonly seen in Alzheimer's patients. This research is still in its infancy, however.

Other Names

- Noopeptide
- GVS-111
- N-phenylacetyl-L-prolylglycine ethyl ester

Type

- Not technically a racetam, but often grouped with them

Benefits

- Enhanced memory
- Improved mood
- Reduced anxiety
- Advanced logical thinking
- Increased creativity
- Better overall cognitive performance

Side Effects/Warnings

The vast majority of Noopept users do not experience any side effects. At the recommended dosages, Noopept has been deemed safe in clinical trials. Symptoms of overdose may include headache, insomnia, fatigue, nausea, and gastrointestinal problems.

Dosage

The recommended starting dosage for Noopept is 10 mg, taken up to 3 times a day. Some people report good results with this dosage. Others require a higher dosage to experience Noopept's benefits. Up to 40 mg per dose seems to be safe and effective for most people. You should always start with a low dose and work your way up as needed.

Some of the effects of Noopept can be felt within a couple of hours after taking it. However, many people report that the full benefits of Noopept don't appear until after several weeks of daily use.

Noopept can be taken with or without food. Taking it on an empty stomach may help it to absorb better. However, some people report mild nausea when taking Noopept on an empty stomach. This is easily remedied by taking it with food.

Oxiracetam

Oxiracetam is a potent nootropic that is one of the more powerful members of the racetam family. It's more powerful than the prototypical racetam, piracetam.

This powerful nootropic has been shown to improve memory, focus, learning, and technical thinking. It also acts as a mild stimulant. Unlike some newer nootropics, oxiracetam has been extensively studied and shown to be safe and effective.

Oxiracetam works in a similar way to the other racetams. It exerts its nootropic benefits by influencing acetylcholine and has been shown to stimulate NDMA and AMPA receptors. Unlike some other racetams, oxiracetam does not seem to influence dopamine, serotonin, or nicotinic receptors.

Other Names

- ISF-2522
- 4-hydroxy-2-oxo-pyrrolidinoacetamide

Type

- Racetam

Benefits

- Increased focus
- Improved memory
- Improved learning
- Increased logical/technical thinking
- Overall cognitive enhancement

Side Effects/Warnings

Side effects are extremely rare with oxiracetam. That is one of the reasons that it is so popular. In several studies, an extremely high dosage was taken by participants for a long period of time. It was shown to be safe, even at high doses for an extended period of time.

A small percentage of people have reported oxiracetam side effects. These included headache, nausea, dizziness, insomnia, irritability, and gastrointestinal distress. Most of these side effects are due to taking oxiracetam on an empty stomach or taking it without a choline source. If you experience nausea or gastrointestinal distress, try taking oxiracetam with food. Headaches and dizziness can usually be avoided by taking oxiracetam with a choline source.

If you are taking the drug carbamazepine, you should not take oxiracetam. Carbamazepine is an anti-convulsant and a mood stabilizer that is commonly used to treat bipolar disorder and other conditions. It has been shown to have an interaction with oxiracetam. This drug interaction is not life threatening and only results in minor side effects.

Dosage

Oxiracetam is typically taken in dosages ranging from 600 to 1,800 mg. You should start with a low dosage and work your way up as needed. Some people get good results with 600 mg, while others require higher dosages to experience oxiracetam's benefits.

For maximum absorption, oxiracetam should be taken on an empty stomach. This may cause nausea in some people. If this occurs, it can be taken with food. A higher dosage may be required to get the desired results.

You should also consider taking a choline source with oxiracetam. If you don't have optimal choline levels, you might not experience its full benefits. Also, taking a choline source with oxiracetam reduces the risk of certain side effects, like headaches and dizziness.

Panax Ginseng

Panax ginseng is a plant that grows naturally in Korea, China, and eastern Asia. It's also known as Korean ginseng, Asian ginseng, or "True Ginseng." Some people refer to it as True Ginseng because it has been studied more than any other type and is a true member of the ginseng genus of plants. Siberian ginseng, for example, seems to have many of the same benefits of Panax ginseng, but belongs to a different genus. American ginseng is a member of the same genus as Panax ginseng and is known to have its own benefits, but has not been studied nearly as much.

Used all over the world for its immune-boosting, cognition-enhancing, stress-reducing, and energy-increasing properties, Panax ginseng has been extensively studied and shown to be very safe. It is considered an adaptogen, because of its ability to help the body and mind deal with stress. Panax ginseng is typically used in pill or capsule form, extracted from the root of the plant. It can also be found in powder form and is a common ingredient in many energy drinks, teas, and special coffees.

Other Names

- True Ginseng
- Ginseng
- Panax
- Wild Ginseng
- Asian Ginseng
- Mountain Ginseng
- Korean Ginseng

Type

- Adaptogen

Benefits

- Improved cognitive performance
- Increased calmness
- Improved mood
- Reduced stress
- Improved quality of life

Side Effects/Warnings

Most people that use Panax ginseng do not report any serious side effects. However, like any time you put anything in your body, side effects are possible. Potential side effects of Panax ginseng may include insomnia, restlessness, anxiety, euphoria, diarrhea, vomiting, headache, nose bleed, breast pain, and hypertension.

Panax ginseng may interact with certain drugs. If you take medication for high blood pressure or are on blood thinners, make sure to talk with your doctor before taking any type of ginseng. Also, if you are pregnant, you should not take Panax ginseng.

Dosage

Dosages ranging from 200 mg to 3,000 mg a day have been shown to be effective. Typically, most people report a noticeable effect from 500 mg and up. This is a good starting dose to see how well it works for you. If you don't get the results you want, you may consider increasing the dosage.

Panax ginseng may be taken with or without food. However, taking it with a meal may increase absorption and reduce the possibility of causing nausea and upset stomach.

Phenylpiracetam

Phenylpiracetam is a powerful nootropic that can improve memory, focus, motivation, and mood. It has been extensively studied and has been shown to be both safe and effective.

It was developed in Russia during the early 1980's. Russian scientists created phenylpiracetam by adding a phenyl group to the well-known drug, piracetam. They found that, by doing this, they had created a compound that was much more potent than piracetam. In fact, it is estimated to be as much as 60 times more potent than piracetam.

Phenylpiracetam is available without a prescription in the United States. However, it is only available in Russia and several European counties with a prescription. It is sold there under then names Carphedon and Phenotropil.

It is so effective at improving mental and physical performance that it has been banned by the World Anti-Doping Agency (WADA). They don't go around banning worthless supplements: They only ban things that work and, for many people, phenylpiracetam works wonders.

Other Names

- Phenotropil
- Carphedon
- (RS)-2-(2-oxo-4-phenylpyrrolidin-1-yl)acetamide
- Fonturacetam

Type

- Racetam

Benefits

- Increased focus
- Improved mood
- Improved memory
- Increased motivation
- Improved physical performance
- Increased alertness
- Increased ability to learn

Side Effects/Warnings

Phenylpiracetam is generally well tolerated and most people don't experience any side effects. It has been extensively studied around the world and is generally considered to be safe.

However, some people do experience side effects. Though rare, this can include headaches, nausea, irritability, insomnia, and gastrointestinal problems. Most of these problems can be avoided or resolved by changing the way you take phenylpiracetam. Taking a choline source, like Alpha GPC, will usually get rid of headaches. If you experience nausea and gastrointestinal distress, try taking phenylpiracetam with food. And if you experience insomnia, reduce your dosage or take it earlier in the day.

Dosage

The recommended phenylpiracetam dosage is anywhere from 100-600 mg a day. You should always start at the low end of this range and work your way up as needed. Many people have great results with between 100-200 mg a day.

It is recommended that you take phenylpiracetam with a choline source. One of the neurotransmitters that phenylpiracetam works on is acetylcholine. By taking phenylpiracetam with a choline source, you ensure that your brain has enough of this neurotransmitter. This will boost the effectiveness of phenylpiracetam and may help to reduce some potential side effects.

Phenylpiracetam is water soluble. Most people report that it works best when it's taken on an empty stomach. However, if you experience nausea when doing this, you should take it with food. It will still work, but you may need a higher phenylpiracetam dosage to get the desired results.

Piracetam

This interesting substance was responsible for starting the entire nootropics movement. Piracetam was first created in 1964 by the Romanian chemist and psychologist, Corneliu E. Giurgea. He was the first person to use the term "nootropic," after noticing piracetam's apparent cognition-enhancing properties. This made piracetam the first nootropic.

In the United States, piracetam is sold as a dietary supplement. In other parts of the world, it's used as a prescription medication to treat a number of conditions. It is used in much of Europe, Russia, South America, and other parts of the world.

Piracetam affects neuronal, vascular, and cognitive function without acting as a stimulant or a sedative. It's a positive allosteric modulator of AMPA receptors. Piracetam also improves the function of the neurotransmitter acetylcholine, which is known to play a role in memory and learning, among other things. Although piracetam is chemically similar to GABA, it does not seem to affect GABA metabolism or GABA receptors.

Other Names

- Nootropil
- Lucetam
- 2-oxo-1-pyrrolidine acetamide
- Pyracetam
- Pyrrolidone Acetamide
- Memotopril
- UCB6215

Type

- Racetam

Benefits

- Improved learning
- Enhanced memory
- Improved mood
- Increased focus
- Reduced anxiety
- Increased sensory perception
- Increased motivation

Side Effects/Warnings

Piracetam has been found to be very well tolerated. Side effects are rare and, when they do happen, are easily reversible by simply discontinuing supplementation.

The side effects that are occasionally reported include excitability, anxiety, insomnia, irritability, headache, agitation, tremor, and hyperkinesia. These have all been reported in studies done on unhealthy and elderly populations.

Some of the potential side effects of piracetam can be eliminated by taking it with a choline source. There is a lot of anecdotal evidence to suggest that taking a choline source with piracetam will increase its effectiveness and reduce unwanted side effects.

Dosage

The standard dosage of piracetam is between 1,200-4,800 mg a day. This should be taken in divided doses, split throughout the day. Most users report good results by splitting it between 2 or 3 doses spaced evenly throughout the day.

Taking a choline source with piracetam is reported to increase its effectiveness and reduce unwanted side effects. Acetylcholine is one of the neurotransmitters that piracetam is known to affect.

Piracetam can be taken with or without food. It is probably absorbed better when taken on an empty stomach. However, if you experience nausea, vomiting, or upset stomach, you should take piracetam with food.

Pramiracetam

This is a potent nootropic and another member of the racetam family. It is one of the most powerful racetams. In fact, it is between 15 and 30 times stronger than the prototypical racetam, piracetam.

Unlike many of the nootropics in the racetam family, pramiracetam exerts its nootropic effects without affecting mood or anxiety levels. It does this by influencing glutamate and acetylcholine receptor sites in the brain. These receptors are known to play an important role in memory, focus, learning, and other cognitive processes.

Many nootropics in the racetam family influence dopamine and serotonin receptors. These receptors are known to play a role in mood, anxiety, sleep, and appetite, among other things. Pramiracetam does not seem to affect these receptors. This explains why it is able to provide cognitive benefits without affecting emotions.

In several countries, pramiracetam is only available with a prescription. It's sold under a few different trade names, including Remen, Neupramir, and Pramistar. In the United States, pramiracetam is available as a dietary supplement.

Other Names

- CI-879
- Diisoprop-yl-(2-oxopyrrolidin-1-yl)acetamide
- Remen
- Pramistar
- Neupramir

Type

- Racetam

Benefits

- Enhanced focus
- Improved working/long-term memory
- Increased learning
- Advanced logical/technical thinking
- Higher sensory perception
- Overall improved cognition

Side Effects/Warnings

Pramiracetam is generally well-tolerated and has few side effects at the recommended dosage. However, side effects can occur. Some of the more common pramiracetam side effects include headache, fatigue, insomnia, nervousness, and gastrointestinal distress.

Many of these side effects can be avoided by doing two things. First, make sure you take a choline source with pramiracetam. And second, take it with food. For the small percentage of people that experience side effects, doing these two things often reduces or eliminates side effects.

Dosage

The recommended pramiracetam dosage is between 200 and 400 mg. It is recommended that you start with 200 mg and work your way up as needed. Many people report great results with a low dosage.

Pramiracetam is fat soluble. It is absorbed best when taken with food, particularly food that contains fat. For maximum absorption, take pramiracetam with a small meal containing between 10 and 15 grams of fat.

It is also suggested that you take pramiracetam with a choline source. If you don't have adequate choline levels, you won't get the full benefits of pramiracetam. Also, taking a choline source with pramiracetam will reduce the chances of some side effects, like headaches.

Rhodiola Rosea

Rhodiola rosea is an herb in the Crassulaceae family of plants. It grows naturally all over the world in cold climates and at high altitudes.

It has a long history of use in traditional Chinese, Russian, and Scandinavian medicine. Practitioners of these early forms of medicine recognized that this powerful plant has anti-fatigue and adaptogenic properties.

More recently, rhodiola rosea has become popular as a dietary supplement. Its users are reporting multiple health and nootropic benefits. Unlike many other supplements, there is actually a good amount of scientific research to support some of the health claims that users are reporting.

Studies have shown that rhodiola rosea can improve mood and well-being, reduce fatigue, improve physical performance, improve cognitive performance, and reduce anxiety. People that use rhodiola for its nootropic properties report all of these benefits and more.

Other Names

- Golden Root
- Rose Root
- Aaron's Rod
- Arctic Root
- King's Crown
- Rosavin
- Orpin Rose
- Rosenroot
- Rhodiola Rhizome

Type

- Adaptogen

Benefits

- Improved mood
- Decreased anxiety
- Improved physical performance
- Improved cognitive performance
- Reduced stress
- Improved sense of well-being
- Increased energy
- Reduced fatigue
- Improved athletic performance
- Improved sleep

Side Effects/Warnings

For most people, rhodiola rosea has very few side effects or none at all. In all the studies we looked at, no serious side effects were reported. The side effects that were reported were mild and uncommon.

Side effects could include dry mouth, nausea, upset stomach, headache, insomnia, and weight loss. A few users have reported slight changes in blood pressure. However, a study that looked at some of the physical effects of rhodiola rosea found that it does not influence blood pressure.

You should use caution if you are taking a monoamine oxidase inhibitor (MAOI). Although we could not find any reports of adverse effects, this combination could potentially lead to a condition called serotonin syndrome, as rhodiola rosea is known to increase serotonin levels.

Dosage

As rhodiola rosea is a plant, different brands will have different concentrations of the active ingredient. You want to use one that has at least 1% salidroside, minimum. Ideally, you want to use one that has 3% salidroside.

When taken daily to prevent fatigue, dosages as low as 50 mg a day may be effective. However, most of the studies that we looked at used much higher dosages.

In the studies that reported the greatest benefits to mood, anxiety, physical performance, and cognition, dosages anywhere from 300-800 mg per day were used. No additional benefits seem to come from taking more than 1,000 mg a day.

Most rhodiola rosea supplements come in 500 mg capsules. Again, you want to use one that ideally has 3% salidroside. If you are using 500 mg capsules, taking one every day may be enough to experience the benefits of this amazing herb. If after a few weeks you still haven't noticed the desired effects, you may want to consider increasing to one capsule twice-a-day.

It shouldn't matter much if you take rhodiola rosea with or without food. It may absorb a little better if taken on an empty stomach. If you experience nausea and upset stomach after taking it on an empty stomach, taking it with a small meal may reduce or eliminate these side effects.

Sulbutiamine

This nootropic is a variation of thiamine (vitamin B1). It was developed in Japan to be a more effective version of vitamin B1. Thiamine was the first B vitamin to be discovered, which is why it's called B1.

Sulbutiamine is able to cross the blood-brain barrier much more efficiently than thiamine. Because of this, sulbutiamine offers all the benefits of thiamine and many more. Thiamine is essential to the biosynthesis of acetylcholine and gamma-aminobutyric acid (GABA). These neurotransmitters are involved in learning, anxiety, and relaxation.

Nootropic users have been using sulbutiamine for its ability to reduce anxiety and improve mood without causing sedation, like many prescription drugs do. Some people actually report a slight stimulating effect. Sulbutiamine is also popular with athletes, as they report it can increase power and reduce recovery time after intense exercise.

The antidepressant effects of sulbutiamine seem to be very powerful for some people. It's thought that this is due to its ability to stimulate the neurotransmitter dopamine, particularly at the D1 receptor site. Unfortunately, these effects seem to diminish over time with recurrent use. For this reason, it should not be used as a primary antidepressant. However, it can certainly be a powerful tool to improve mood if used occasionally.

Sulbutiamine has also been shown to improve memory in scientific studies. This isn't surprising, as it boosts the neurotransmitters dopamine and acetylcholine, which are known to play a role in memory, learning, attention, motivation, and pleasure.

Other Names

- Arcalion
- Enerion
- Bisibuthiamine
- Youvitan

Type

- Misc/Other

Benefits

- Improved mood
- Reduced anxiety
- Improved memory
- Improved stamina and endurance

Side Effects/Warnings

Most people seem to tolerate sulbutiamine well. Side effects are rarely reported. When side effects are reported, it's usually because the recommended dosage was exceeded. Side effects can include anxiety, irritability, depression, headaches, nausea, and skin rash. If you experience any side effects, they should go away as soon as you stop using sulbutiamine.

Dosage

The recommended sulbutiamine dosage is between 500 and 1,000 mg. It is generally recommended that you start with a lower dose to see how it affects you. Many people experience the benefits of sulbutiamine with just 500 mg.

Sulbutiamine is fat soluble. Because of this, you should take it with food that contains 10-15 grams of fat. This will help your body absorb more of this potent nootropic.

Sunifiram

This is a relatively new nootropic that has been getting some attention in the nootropics community over the past couple years. Although there hasn't been much research on it yet, preliminary studies are very promising. Users from around the world are reporting that sunifiram has a number of potent nootropic and mood-boosting properties.

Sunifiram is a synthetic derivative of piracetam, which is one of the the world's oldest and best-studied nootropics. It's significantly more potent than piracetam, so a much lower dosage is needed to experience sunifiram's benefits. While piracetam doses are measured in grams, sunifiram doses are measured in single-digit milligrams.

Sunifiram is known as an ampakine because its main mechanism of action is via the AMPA receptor. AMPA is one of the three main subsets of glutamate receptors, along with NDMA and kainate. Sunifiram is a positive allosteric modulator of AMPA and it activates AMPA-mediated neurotransmission. It has also been shown to aid in the release of acetylcholine in the cerebral cortex. As you know, acetylcholine plays a role in learning, memory, decision making, and many other cognitive processes.

While sunifiram is a derivative of the racetamic nootropic piracetam, it is not technically a racetam itself. This is because sunifiram does not have the same chemical (pyrrolidone) backbone that piracetam and all the other racetams have. Sunifiram is chemically similar to other piperazine alkaloids, such as unifiram and sapunifiram.

Other Names

- DM-235

Type

- Not technically a racetam, but derived from one

Benefits

- Improved memory
- Increased focus
- Improved mood
- Improved decision making
- Improved overall cognitive function
- Increased alertness
- Increased feeling of well-being

Side Effects/Warnings

There have not been any human studies done on the long-term safety of sunifiram. However, due to sunifiram's structural and functional similarities to other nootropics, we can reasonably assume that it has a similar safety profile.

No serious side effects have ever been reported with sunifiram. Some users report over-stimulation, insomnia, and anxiety when using extremely high doses (> 12 mg). This can easily be avoided by staying within the recommended dosing range.

Two of the most common side effects seen with sunifiram and many other nootropics are headaches and upset stomach. Both of these potential side effects can usually be reduced or eliminated. If you experience upset stomach when taking sunifiram, try taking it with a small meal. This eliminates nausea and upset stomach for most users.

It is also a good idea to take a choline source with sunifiram. Some users of sunifiram and several other nootropics report getting headaches. This is thought to be caused by changes in acetylcholine levels in the brain. By taking a choline source, you ensure that you have adequate levels of acetylcholine, thus reducing the likelihood of headaches.

Dosage

Sunifiram is an extremely potent nootropic, so you only need a small amount to experience big effects. While there have been no human studies done to figure out the optimal sunifiram dosage, we can look at animal studies and the dozens of case reports published online to come up with an effective dosing range.

An effective sunifiram dosage for most people seems to be between 5 and 10 mg. At the lower end of this range, users report an increase in focus, memory, and overall cognitive function. At the higher end and beyond, users often report more of a stimulating effect, in addition to all the effects felt at lower dosages.

As always, it's recommended that you start at the lower end of this range and work your way up as needed. Many users get the results they want with only 5 mg of sunifiram.

Vinpocetine

This is a nootropic that has tons of potential benefits. This interesting supplement can improve cognition, mood, hearing, vision, cardiovascular health, and has anti-inflammatory effects. One of the more interesting uses of vinpocetine is for the treatment of tinnitus (ringing in the ears). This is a problem that affects many people and its causes are poorly understood. A lot of people that suffer from tinnitus have reported that vinpocetine supplementation improved their symptoms significantly.

Vinpocetine is extracted from the periwinkle plant. It was first discovered in 1975. By 1978, it was already being used for its many medical benefits.

In some European countries, vinpocetine is only available with a prescription. It is prescribed there for a wide variety of medical and psychological conditions. In the United States, it is sold as a dietary supplement and can be purchased without a prescription.

Other Names

- Vincamine
- Vinca Minor
- Periwinkle Extract
- Cavinton
- Ethyl Apovincaminate
- Intelectol

Type

- Misc/Other

Benefits

- Improved memory
- Increased learning
- Improved hearing function
- Improved vision
- Improved cardiovascular function

Side Effects/Warnings

Vinpocetine is generally well tolerated. In clinical trials, no serious side effects were reported. Some users report headaches and upset stomach with higher doses. This can usually be avoided by taking vinpocetine with a choline source and by taking it with food.

Dosage

The recommended dosage for vinpocetine is between 10 and 30 mg. You should always start with a low dose and work your way up as needed. Some people experience all of vinpocetine's benefits with only 10 mg.

It is generally recommended that you take vinpocetine with food. This will not only help to reduce the possibility of nausea and upset stomach, but it will also help it absorb better.

Other Nootropics

The nootropics listed above are some of the safest, most effective, and most commonly used. However, there are tons of other substances that people use to improve brain function. Here's a list of some other popular nootropics you can look into on your own, if you're interested:

- Armodafinil
- Bromantane
- Centrophenoxine
- Choline Bitartrate
- Fasoracetam
- Hordenine
- Huperzine-A
- Insulin (used nasally)
- Kratom
- Nefiracetam
- PEA (Phenyethylamine)
- Picamilon
- Selank
- Selegiline
- Semax
- Tianeptine
- Tyrosine
- Unifiram
- Uridine

CHAPTER FIVE

Stacking Nootropics

What is a "stack?"

Stacking supplements is nothing new. It's been a common part of sports nutrition and performance enhancement for a long time. And for the past few years, it has been commonly seen with cognitive enhancement, too.

"Stacking" simply means to take more than one substance at a time. This is done primarily to improve results and reduce side effects. Many nootropics work better when taken in combinations. These combinations are usually referred to as "stacks."

Is it safe to stack nootropics?

Most people that take multiple nootropics at a time don't experience any serious side effects. However, negative interactions can occasionally occur.

You should always do your research before stacking nootropics. Make sure there are no known interactions between them. For example, you generally should not stack multiple stimulants together, as this can put a dangerous strain on your cardiovascular system.

That being said, most nootropics do stack well together. Since everyone's brains are different, each person may find that certain stacks work better for them than for others. To find out what your optimal nootropic stack is, you may have to be willing to experiment on yourself a little bit.

A lot of companies have been coming out with pre-made nootropic stacks over the past couple years. As the popularity of nootropics continues to grow, more and more will surely hit the market.

The problem with these pre-made formulas is that, since everyone's brains are different, not everyone is gonna respond to them the same. In fact, few people respond to pre-made stacks at all. And another big problem with them is the price. It's much cheaper to purchase individual nootropics to make your own stacks than to buy ones that are already made. So, in other words, stay away from pre-made formulas.

3 nootropic stacks for beginners

Here are 3 basic stacks that are excellent for anyone that is new to the wonderful world of cognitive enhancement. These stacks were chosen because they're safe, effective, and simple. But just because these stacks are ideal for beginners, doesn't mean that they aren't still popular with more experienced users. Nootropic users of all experience levels can and do use these powerful combinations.

Caffeine and L-Theanine

This is a very basic nootropic stack. It's also a very popular stack and for good reason: It works. It's no secret that caffeine can improve focus, increase wakefulness, and give you a little mood boost. But those effects sometimes come at a price: increased anxiety and an uncomfortable jittery feeling. Taking l-theanine with caffeine can help to strip away those unwanted side effects, leaving you feeling awake and focused, yet relaxed and calm at the same time.

Most people that use the caffeine and l-theanine stack find that a 1:2 ratio works best. So, for every 100 mg of caffeine, you'd take 200 mg of l-theanine. The most common dosage used is 200 mg of caffeine and 400 mg of l-theanine. Some users find that using as much as 500 mg of caffeine and 1,000 mg (1g) of l-theanine is optimal. However, you should start with a low dosage to begin with and go from there. If you don't get the results you want with a lower dosage, gradually increase it until you find the dose that works best for you.

Benefits of caffeine and l-theanine:

- Increased focus
- Reduced anxiety
- Improved mood
- Promotes a calm, focused mindset
- Improved learning
- Promotes a feeling of relaxed alertness

The caffeine and l-theanine stack is considered to be very safe. Most users report no side effects. However, any of the usual side effects of caffeine can occur, although are less likely because of the l-theanine. This stack works best when taken on an empty stomach but, if you experience upset stomach, it may be taken with food.

Noopept and Choline

This is another popular and effective nootropic stack. Noopept is a well-known nootropic that is often suggested as a first nootropic. That's because it's safe, effective, and less expensive than many other nootropics. But if you just take Noopept by itself, you could be missing out on some of its benefits.

Noopept works on several neurotransmitters, one of which is acetylcholine. If your acetylcholine levels aren't optimized, you won't get all the benefits of Noopept. The obvious solution is to take a choline source with it.

There are a number of different choline sources available. The two that are most often used are alpha-GPC and CDP-choline. Stacking a choline source with Noopept ensures that your acetylcholine levels are high enough to reap the full benefits of this powerful nootropic.

Benefits of Noopept and choline:

- Improved cognitive performance
- Reduced anxiety
- Improved mood
- Increased creativity
- Enhanced memory
- Advanced logical thinking

Noopept and choline users have reported positive effects from a variety of different dosages. Typically, Noopept is taken at a dosage of 10, 20, or 30 mg, up to three times a day. Some users report much high dosages, but this is not recommended. The dosage of choline will depend on what type of choline you're using. If you're using alpha-GPC, a typical dose would be anywhere from 500 mg to 1,500 mg a day. The dosage for CDP-choline is similar, ranging from 500 mg to 2,000 mg a day, taken in one or more doses.

Piracetam, Oxiracetam, and Alpha-GPC

Our third and final stack contains 3 different nootropics: piracetam, oxiracetam, and alpha-GPC. Like the stacks above, this combination has been used safely and effectively by countless nootropic users. Let's look at each of these nootropics and what they contribute to the stack.

Piracetam – This is the one that started it all. Piracetam was the drug that inspired the creation of the word "nootropic." It's been around for a long time, has an excellent safety profile, and can be very effective. Piracetam can improve learning, enhance memory, improve mood, increase motivation, and even reduce anxiety. It can be highly effective on its own, but taking it with a choline source (like alpha-GPC) can make it even more so. Piracetam is the backbone of this simple, powerful stack.

Oxiracetam – Like piracetam, oxiracetam is also in the racetam family of nootropics. Oxiracetam is effective and has an excellent safety record. It's been shown to improve focus, memory, and learning without affecting mood or anxiety. Adding oxiracetam to this stack will add to piracetam's ability to improve focus, memory, and learning.

Alpha-GPC – The last nootropic in this stack is our choline source, alpha-GPC. There are several different choline sources but we picked alpha-GPC because it fits with the rest of this stack: It's safe, effective, and affordable. Alpha-GPC increases levels of acetylcholine, making piracetam and oxiracetam more effective.

Benefits of piracetam, oxiracetam, and alpha-GPC:

- Improved learning
- Improved memory
- Increased focus
- Improved mood
- Reduced anxiety
- Overall cognitive enhancement

It would be wise to start with the lowest recommended dosage of each nootropic and increase them as necessary. That would mean 1,200 mg of piracetam, 600 mg of oxiracetam, and 500 mg of alpha-GPC. Some users report amazing benefits from these low dosages and never need to increase them. Others notice little effect and have to increase the dosage of each to get the benefits they want. Everyone is different, so you may have to experiment a bit to figure out what works best for you.

While most nootropics can be used on their own, many users find that they're more effective when stacked together. Most people will experience at least some benefit for these three stacks. However, everyone's brains are wired differently, so not everyone responds the same way to the same things. You may have to experiment on yourself a little bit to see what works best for you.

CHAPTER SIX

Where To Buy Nootropics

Just a few short years ago, there were only a few nootropic suppliers in the world. Now, there are dozens and dozens of companies that sell them and more popping up every day.

We're gonna list a few of the best places to buy nootropics online and where to find certain nootropics offline. These companies all have excellent products, reasonable prices, fast shipping, and great customer service.

However, since new nootropic companies are popping up regularly, this list will be constantly changing. If you want see an updated list of the best places to buy nootropics, go to the Nootropics Zone website (www.nootropicszone.com) and click "Where To Buy Nootropics" at the top.

Online retailers

Nootropics City

Nootropics City has become one of our favorite all-around companies to buy nootropics and other brain supplements from. They've really separated themselves from the competition over the past couple years. We really can't say enough good things about them.

The first thing that you'll notice is that they have an absolutely amazing selection of all the most popular nootropics. They also carry a few that are hard to find.

Second, you'll notice that most of the nootropics they have are in pill or capsule form. This is important for a lot of people. Many nootropic users, especially new users, don't want to deal with measuring out powders. Pills and capsules are much easier to use.

Third, their customer service is top notch. We've had conversations with several employees/owners at Nootropics City and their commitment to making their customers happy is very apparent.

Fourth, fifth, and sixth: they have reasonable prices, fast shipping, and all their products are of the highest quality and purity. We've been ordering from them for a long time and will continue to do so. We've never had anything but great experiences with Nootropics City. Very highly recommended.

Absorb Health

This is a great company that sells a variety of nootropics and other supplements. Almost all of the noots that they sell are in capsule form, which is what a lot of people are looking for. Their prices are reasonable, have fast shipping, good customer service, and all of their products seem to be very high quality.

We've ordered from Absorb Health many times and will continue to in the future. They have a large selection of other supplements too, in addition to their impressive nootropic selection. We always recommend Absorb Health to anyone that is new to the world of smart drugs. Their website is easy to use and they carry all of the nootropics that are usually recommended for first-time users.

Peak Nootropics

We've been using these guys for a couple years now and can't say enough good things about them. For a long time, they only had powders, but they have recently added a number of nootropics in capsule form.

Peak nootropics offer a diverse selection of nootropics. They carry all of the usual noots, like most of the common racetams and choline sources. But they also have some of the newer and rarer nootropics like coluracetam and sunifiram.

Their customer service is very good, their prices are reasonable, and their shipping is fast. Peak Nootropics is a great place for intermediate-level nootropic users.

Powder City

Guess what these guys carry the most of? That's right, you guessed it: Powders. These guys have a very impressive selection of supplements in powder form. They also carry a number of capsules. But, as their name implies, most of their products are in powder form.

We've only used Powder City a couple of times but both our experiences were positive. Their products are very high quality and they ship pretty fast. They carry a few powders that can't be found at any of the other nootropic vendors.

We generally only use these guys for things that we can't get from the above vendors. Their prices are good and they have a large selection of other, non-nootropic supplements. This supplier is probably best for more experienced users. Some of the products they sell in powder form can be dangerous, if misused.

Duck Dose

The last nootropic supplier on our list is Duck Dose. This company is relatively new but have already proven themselves to be a reliable seller. Duck Dose only sells two nootropics: modafinil and armodafinil. We've decided to include them on our list of where to buy nootropics because none of the other vendors on the list sell these two powerful nootropics.

Duck Dose carries pharmaceutical grade modafinil and armodafinil, manufactured by two different companies. The quality of their products is excellent (again, pharma-grade), their customer service is amazing, and their shipping is fast and discreet.

But again, make sure to check out the Nootropic Zone's "Where To Buy Nootropics" post for an updated list and links to all these vendors' secure websites.

Nootropics sold in stores

Some nootropics can be found in offline, brick-and-mortar stores. Places like Wal Mart and other large department stores, pharmacies, and supplement shops all carry some nootropics.

The selection and quality that you'll find will be very limited, though. Generally, the only nootropics that you're likely to find in stores are caffeine, l-theanine, ginkgo biloba, ginseng, and maybe one or two others. We've never seen any racetams, eugeroics, cholinergics, or other nootropics in any stores.

CHAPTER SEVEN

Where To Go From Here

Now that you know all about nootropics, where do you go from here? In this chapter, we're gonna discuss trying your first nootropic, where to learn even more about nootropics, and keeping track of your results.

But before we do that, we're gonna talk about how to boost cognitive performance without drugs. For nootropics to work optimally, there are a few things you need to take care of first. Let's go over those things now.

How to *really* improve cognitive performance

If you want to *really* improve cognitive function, don't look to nootropics – not yet, anyway. First, you need to make sure you're doing all the things we're gonna talk about here. Every single nootropic will work better if you follow this advice.

Will they work if you don't? Sure, most of them will. But they won't work as well as they could. This is *your* brain, *your* body, and *your* life – You should be willing to do whatever it takes to get the most out of it.

These things won't cost you anything, yet are worth more than all the nootropics in the world. Before you start taking smart drugs, you should make sure you're doing all of the following.

Exercise

"What does exercise have to do with boosting cognitive function?" you may be asking. Honestly, it has everything to do with it. If you aren't currently getting regular exercise, adding 30-45 minutes a day will do more for your cognitive performance than any pill, powder, plant, or potion.

It's no secret that exercise is good for the heart and the rest of the cardiovascular system. But it's also essential for optimal brain function. Numerous studies have shown that regular exercise can increase neurological activity, improve memory, enhance cognitive control of behavior, reduce stress, and improve mood. And, as if that's not enough, regular exercise will help you build muscle and burn fat. Feeling better about the way you look will improve confidence and self-esteem, which can also indirectly improve cognition.

If you're not getting at least 30 minutes of moderate-to-intense physical activity every day, you're doing your body and brain a disservice. And, if you're serious about improving cognitive function, exercise will do more for your brain than any nootropic. That's because exercise has been shown to influence many of the same neurotransmitters that nootropics do. If you really want to improve cognitive function, make sure you're getting plenty of exercise.

Nutrition

It's no secret that what you eat has a direct impact on the way your body looks, works, and feels. If you eat more calories than your body uses every day over a period of time, you'll gain weight. If you don't get enough vitamins and minerals, you'll develop a deficiency. And if you eat too much sugar for too long, you can develop diabetes.

We're all aware of examples like these and know that our diets directly affect our bodies. But what you might not know is that our diets have a direct impact on cognitive function. You've probably noticed that when you get really hungry, it's harder to concentrate and your mood dips a bit. Or, like most people, you're well-aware of the "crash" that occurs a few hours after consuming coffee or high-sugar snacks. These are examples of acute changes in cognitive function that are directly related to what we eat. But, our diets also affect how we think and feel over long periods of time, too.

If you want to really improve cognitive function, you need to make sure you're getting the proper nutrition to optimize brain function. What does this mean, exactly? Well, exact nutritional needs vary from person to person, but we'll go over the basic things needed for optimal brain health.

Staying properly hydrated is one of the most important things you can do for your brain. When you become even mildly dehydrated, your visual-motor tracking decreases, short-term memory becomes impaired, ability to concentrate decreases, and subjective well-being declines. Make sure you're drinking plenty of water throughout the day to avoid becoming dehydrated.

Another important way to optimize brain health is by making sure you're getting all the vitamins and minerals (micronutrients) that your body needs. As many as 90% of Americans do not get the recommended daily amount of vitamins and minerals. Vitamin deficiencies can significantly impair just about every aspect of cognition. The best way to make sure you're getting all the micronutrients that your body and brain needs is to regularly eat a variety of fruits and vegetables. If you can't get all of your vitamins and minerals from food, taking a daily multivitamin can help you make sure you're getting all the micronutrients that you need.

Lastly, you should try to eat a well-balanced diet and limit your sugar, saturated and trans fats, and sodium intake. A well-balanced diet includes lean meats, fruits and vegetables, whole grains, and low-fat dairy products. Excess sugar, saturated fat and trans fats, and sodium can all have a negative impact on your cognitive functioning.

Nutrition is a fascinating and complicated subject that we can't fully explore here. But, if you follow the basic advice above, you'll be giving your brain everything it needs to function optimally.

Sleep

The last thing you need to do to really improve cognitive function is make sure you're getting enough good-quality sleep. If you're not getting enough sleep or you are but often wake up without feeling rested, you're not alone: 45% of Americans report that poor or insufficient sleep has affected the quality of their lives within the past week. Even mild sleep deprivation is known to impair short and long-term memory, attention, focus, vigilance, and several other aspects of cognitive functioning. It's extremely important that you get enough good-quality sleep for optimal brain function.

You've probably heard that you need 8 hours of sleep every night. While this may be true for some people, it's certainly not true for everyone. Different people require different amounts of sleep to function optimally. Some people thrive on 6 hours of sleep per night. Others feel tired all day if they get anything less than 10 hours. No one can tell you what the optimal amount of sleep is for you. Everyone's brains and bodies are unique and require different amounts of rest.

If you feel like you're not getting enough sleep, improving your diet and exercising daily can make a major difference. Going to sleep at the same time every night, limiting caffeine and other stimulants late in the day, and having a consistent sleep ritual can all help you get the rest that your body needs.

As a last resort, after you've improved your diet and increased your physical activity level, you may want to consider taking medication or supplements if you still aren't getting enough sleep. There are a number of prescription medications available that are effective at helping you sleep. Unfortunately, many of them come with unwanted side effects, including morning grogginess.

There are also a variety of supplements that can help with sleep. Melatonin, kava, and valerian are all common supplements that can be used to help you fall asleep and stay asleep. Though they can also have unwanted side effects, most people find that they are much easier to tolerate than prescription drugs.

Your first nootropic

If you've never tried a nootropic before but are now ready to take your brain to the next level, you might be a little overwhelmed by the vast selection of nootropics available. We're gonna list a few nootropics that are safe, effective, and ideal for someone that is new to the wonderful world of smart drugs.

Which nootropic(s) you choose will depend on what effects you're looking for. Maybe you want to improve focus and reduce anxiety. Or perhaps you want something that improves memory without affecting mood or anxiety. Below is a short list of nootropics and nootropic stacks that are ideal for the first-time user.

Caffeine and L-Theanine – This is a perfect beginner stack, ideal for someone looking to induce a state of relaxed focus. All the benefits of caffeine, but with no jitters or anxiety.

Noopept – A great first all-around nootropic. Noopept can improve focus, motivation, mood, and anxiety. It is generally well-tolerated and works great for many people that try it. To reduce the possibility of side effects and increase benefits, stack Noopept with a choline source.

Piracetam – The nootropic that started it all, piracetam has been extensively studied and shown to be both safe and effective. This has been the first nootropic of countless smart drug users. Consider stacking with a choline source to increase effects.

CDP-Choline – This is another great first nootropic, especially if you suffer from brain fog, poor memory, or have trouble concentrating. CDP-choline will raise acetylcholine levels in the brain, resulting in improved focus, memory, and motivation. And, it stacks well with most other nootropics.

Where to learn more

If you're interested in learning more about nootropics, the following resources are a great place to start. It's important that you know where to look for current, accurate information.

The Nootropics Zone – www.nootropicszone.com

Of course we're gonna list our own website here! The Nootropics Zone was created in 2014 with one goal in mind: to provide current, evidence-based information about everything related to nootropics.

When we first started out a few years ago, we were one of the only nootropics websites on the internet. Now, there's dozens and dozens of them. Unfortunately, many of them exist only to make money and don't provide much valuable information - only copywritten articles intended to sell you stuff.

While the Nootropics Zone does make money from affiliate sales (which we've always been upfront about), our articles are all well-researched, referenced, and include both the positives *and* negatives of each nootropic. We want our readers to have access to current and accurate information so they can make informed decisions.

Make sure to check out The Nootropics Zone for all the latest info about smart drugs. And please sign up for our newsletter. We only send out one or two a month (at most) and you'll get a free gift for signing up.

Examine – www.examine.com

This website is an amazing resource for anyone interested in researching specific drugs, supplements, plants, vitamins, minerals, and herbs. Examine has become our go-to for information about nootropics. Just search for whatever nootropic you're interested in and it provides a breakdown of and links to all the evidence.

The thing that makes Examine great is that there are no opinions – just facts. It's a very plain, no-frills website. Examine gives a brief description of each substance, dosage information, a chart of all the effects, a semi-detailed breakdown of all the evidence, and a list of references.

For those of you that are interested in the science behind nootropic use, Examine is an invaluable resource. Everything is meticulously cited. That's why Examine is usually our starting-point when doing nootropics research. It presents all the evidence and provides all the sources, so we can *examine* the data ourselves.

Even if you aren't interested in the science behind nootropics, you may still want to check out Examine. It's a great place for nootropic information. It's actually a great place for information about all kinds of supplements.

LongeCity – www.longecity.com/forums

This is a great website and a great community of people that are interested in nootropics and other areas of personal enhancement. What makes LongeCity an amazing resource is their forum. They have a great forum with topics about all kinds of things directly and indirectly related to smart drugs.

Some of these topics include bioscience, supplements, brain health, lifestyle, biofeedback, spirituality, and medicine. As you can see, these are all related in some way to nootropics.

The thing that really makes this site a great resource for nootropic information is the LongeCity community. It's made up of people from all walks of life, discussing all the things mentioned above and more.

You can read people's personal experiences with specific nootropics or nootropic stacks. If you have questions, you're sure to get quick and informative answers from the community. And it provides a great place to share information with other like-minded individuals.

Reddit – www.reddit.com/r/nootropics/

Another great online nootropics community is Reddit. If you're not familiar with Reddit, it's a gigantic message board-style website where you can make text posts and share links.

Topics covered by Reddit? Everything you can think of. Reddit is organized by topic, which are divided into "subreddits." As of right now, there are over 800,000 subreddits.

If you've never used Reddit, you should check it out. It's a great place to chat with like-minded people, but not just for nootropics info. It's also a great resource for any other interests you may have.

Reddit is a great place to learn about nootropics and to ask questions. Reddit is super easy to use. To sign up, all you need is a user name and a password: That's it – No email address, no real name... nothing. This makes Reddit a great place to ask questions anonymously.

The nootropics community on Reddit is great. It currently has over 80,000 members and is growing rapidly. This community is very active. There are dozens of new posts every day. If you have a question about nootropics, it's likely to get answered quickly – sometimes within minutes.

If you've never used Reddit, it's worth checking out. For nootropic information or info about any other interest you may have, Reddit can be an amazing resource.

Facebook Groups

If we had to guess, we'd guess that you use Facebook. It's a pretty safe bet, since 71% of people in the U.S. do. More than 1.5 billion people use Facebook every month. This number isn't surprising. Facebook is a convenient, easy-to-use place to connect with people and stay up-to-date with current events.

One of the ways that you can connect with like-minded people on Facebook is by joining a group. Facebook has more than half a billion groups. And a handful of these groups are either directly or indirectly related to nootropics.

While there are several nootropic groups on Facebook, there are two that stand out as the best. The first one is called "Better Living Through Nootropics." It's a bit newer than some of the other groups, but its membership is growing quickly.

The other nootropics group we recommend is simply called "Nootropics." This group is much older and has many more members.

These two are the best nootropics groups of Facebook. They both have good content and plenty of active members. Better Living Through Nootropics may be easier to navigate, though, as it doesn't have nearly as many members. Since the other group is so large, it can sometimes be hard to sort through all the content.

These groups are a great place to ask questions, share links, and discuss anything related to nootropics.

Keeping track of your results

Although it's not necessary, you may want to keep a record of the nootropics that you try and the results that you get from them. Some nootropic users, especially those that like to stack multiple smart drugs, find that keeping a log helps them to figure out what combinations work best.

The easiest way to do this is to create a spreadsheet or to simply use a text document. If you do decide to keep track of your nootropic use, you'll want to record some or all of the following details:

- Name of nootropic
- Dosage
- Date and time taken
- Effects
- Side-effects
- How long until the effects were felt
- How long did the effects last
- Any other relevant information

Again, keeping track of your nootropic use isn't necessary but may help you to figure out what works best for you.

CHAPTER EIGHT

Conclusion

Thank you for reading Nootropics: Unlocking Your True Potential With Smart Drugs! You should now have all the information you need to start unlocking *your* true potential.

We tried to include everything that someone new to nootropics would need to know to start benefiting from these wonderful substances. You should now know what they are, how they work, the different types, where to buy, and how to take them.

If there's anything you think we missed or that you'd like to see included in a future edition, please let us know here: feedback@nootropicszone.com.

And lastly, please sign up for the Nootropics Zone newsletter to stay up-to-date with everything going on in the nootropics world. We'll keep you informed about new nootropics, new places to buy them, and all the latest news about smart drugs.

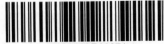

Made in the USA
San Bernardino, CA
02 June 2019